MW00463369

Brain Damage
in Contact Sports

What Parents Should Know
Before Letting Their
Children Play

Dr. Bennet Omalu

MD, MBA, MPH, CPE, DABP-AP, CP, FP, NP
Forensic Pathologist/Neuropathologist/Epidemiologist

Neo-Forenxis Books
Stockton, California

Neo-Forenxis Books

3031 West March Lane, #323,

Stockton, CA 95829

www.bennetomalu.com

Editorial review and revisions performed by Cynthia Chin and Mayapriya Long.

Cover and text design by Mayapriya Long, Bookwrights

Illustrations by Arielle Si

ISBN: 978-0-9916353-2-0

To every parent whose child has suffered
brain damage while playing sports.
My heart is with you.
Your pain is my pain.

Best Wishes

Bennet

Other books by Dr. Bennet I. Omalu

Play Hard, Die Young

*A Historical Foundation of
CTE in Football Players*

Truth Doesn't Have a Side

Contents

Acknowledgments 7

Introduction 9

1. I Care Deeply about Your Child—
and the Truth 11

2. It's Crazy to Tell Me That My Child
Should Not Play Football 21

3. The Brain Floats Like a Balloon inside
the Skull 27

4. Myth: The $1,200 Helmet I Purchased
Will Protect My Child's Brain 35

5. A Blow to the Head, a Sub-Concussion
and a Concussion? 41

6. Brain Damage Caused by Playing
Football Is Real; These Stories
Illustrate It 49

7. What Is CTE and How Is It Different from
Brain Damage? 61

8. If Brain Damage Is This Serious, Then
What the Heck Is the NFL Doing? 73

9. Should Football Be Banned to Protect
   Our Children?. 79

10. Is It Child Abuse to Let My Child Play
    Football? 83

11. Should I Let My Child Play Lacrosse or
    Soccer?. 91

12. Brain Damage Is Not Only about
    Sports 101

13. I Understand, But It Won't Happen to My
    Child 109

Acknowledgments

Arielle Si, thank you so much for your originality and the pristine creativity in your illustrations. Dr. Susan Parson, you inspired me at a challenging time while I wrote this book, and thank you so much for introducing me to Cynthia Chin. For your talent and transparent sincerity, Cynthia Chin I thank you so much. Mayapriya Long, you and I go way back, and you chose to believe in me, when many did not, I am deeply grateful. Prema, Ashly and Mark I love you so very much, and thank you for your patience and tolerance. I will continue to strive to always be a better husband and father. May God continue to bless you all most abundantly.

Introduction

Ever since my discovery of CTE (Chronic Traumatic Encephalopathy) shook the NFL,* and the movie that chronicles my life, *Concussion,* was released, parents across the world have reached out to me, desperately seeking help for their children. Many of them tell me that they were not aware of brain injuries related to football and other contact sports. They tell me that they wish they had known. Over many months of receiving these distressing pleas, I thought of writing a short, heartfelt book for parents about this very topic. You are reading the manifestation of that urging.

My goal in the following pages is to be as logically honest and transparent as I can. It's who I am and how God has made me. I say things as they are. I am not someone one who is politically correct when it comes to traumatic brain injuries and the sports that encourage them. Many other doctors do not want to say what I am about to share with you, especially in print, or in front of the camera. Simply put, they may be afraid.

I am a proud American. I love our country, its traditions, and its beautiful, hardworking people.

---

* For more of my personal story, and the journey of my research and struggle against the NFL, I encourage you to read *Truth Doesn't Have a Side* by Dr. Bennet Omalu with Mark Tabb (Zondervan, 2017).

I have traveled extensively across our nation and have lived on both coasts. However, what I have come to understand about this America that I love, and perhaps the general era in which we live, is that people are willing to deny the truth for convenience. Whatever makes them feel good, is okay. And even if what they tell themselves is a lie that will inevitably harm them, or even cause them to die, that's okay, too. This should not be so.

When you speak the truth, as I am about to, you're bound to offend people who want to believe their own alternative narrative. It is not my wish to offend you. It is my desire to be honest. What I am about to say is controversial and upsetting. But it is truthful, and that is what I stand for.

Like you, I am a parent, and I speak to you as one parent to another, pleading with you to know that my heart and mind are for your child: his/her health, happiness, well-being, intelligence, and the fullness and richness of life that he/she is so richly bestowed as God's creation. This radical honesty just might save your child's life.

After you have read and digested these words that flow from my heart, please search your own. You will know the right thing to do. And I urge you to spread this truth to other parents.

For Truth, and Your Child's Sake,

Dr. Bennet Omalu
Stockton, California

1

I Care Deeply about Your Child—and the Truth

I always wake up early, around 2 to 4 a.m. On one such early Sunday morning, I checked my email to discover that overnight I had received a message from a mother who had two teenage children, a son and a daughter. The son, who we'll call Dan, was about 16 years old and began playing football when he was six. Remarkably gifted, several colleges had already offered him football scholarships. As I read, her email grew fraught with fear. Despite her son's success, this mother recounted observing what at first were only subtle behavioral changes. Over time, Dan had become increasingly impulsive and short-tempered, with rampant mood fluctuations. He was also beginning to become uncharacteristically forgetful, displaying bouts of anger while looking for misplaced items. His performance in school was also beginning to suffer. The mom believed that these changes were merely the excesses of a teenage boy made popular by playing football.

She then described what happened only hours before, which caused her to frantically search for my email address on the internet. The panic in her words was palpable. Dan had lost his temper over some trivial matter at home and violently slapped his little sister twice across the face. As soon as he did, he broke down sobbing, yelling that he did not know what had come over him. This was the first time in the history of this precious family that any type of cruelty had ever taken place.

The poor mother could not sleep all night. "Please help me," she wrote. I could almost see her tears. I replied with a heavy heart, telling her what I would tell every parent: her child should stop playing football immediately.

She replied quickly. In her response to me, you could vividly see her internal struggles and conflicting emotions. While she was afraid for her son and would not want him to suffer brain damage, she was also happy that he was the popular kid in school who seemed to have a bright future as a football star.

But what type of bright future would her son have if he suffers permanent brain damage after spending only three or five years in the NFL (which is about the average span of the career of every professional football player)? With the brain damage he would suffer playing football for decades, what would her son do with the rest of his life after he retired from football in his mid-thirties? If he did not play football and did not suffer any brain damage would he have a better chance to make it in life in his forties, fifties, sixties and afterwards? Undeniably—yes.

More email correspondence revealed that the mom wanted Dan to continue playing so he would make it to the NFL, but she did not want him to suffer any form of brain damage. Sadly, I realized that this was why she reached out to me—she wanted me to somehow do my magic, protect her son and prevent him from suffering any permanent, irreversible damage to his brain. But, the truth will not let her have it both ways.

Other than giving her my sincere advice, there was nothing I could do for her or for her son. I advised her to first, have Dan stop playing football immediately. I also counseled her with the truth that there is nothing any doctor can do for a child once he has suffered brain damage. Even if he had suffered some degree of brain damage at the time she reached out to me, her son could still stop playing immediately in order to prevent more blows to his head and more brain damage.

At some point I stopped responding to her e-mails. I had exhausted all I could do for her. While I struggled to tell her the real truth, she would respond by presenting alternative truths to me that would make her feel better and calm her fears. If Dan continued to play football, his life would be destroyed. Period. It was already happening.

I am a parent, too.

I have two children, Ashly and Mark. Ashly was born two years and five months before Mark. On the day Ashly was born, the nurses bathed and clothed her and placed her in my arms. I stared at her beautifully formed, sleeping face. After a few contented minutes she opened her eyes and looked into mine. At that moment I thought I saw the eyes of God. Tears rolled down my cheeks.

My middle name is Ifeankandu. It means "life is the greatest gift of all." At that moment, looking into the very soul of my precious daughter, my middle name took a new meaning: "the life of my child is the greatest gift of my life." I would now do everything within my power for this little girl—even sacrifice my own life.

I believe every parent feels the same way about his or her child, as I am sure you do, as I'm sure Dan's mom does. As a parent, I know you will do all you can to help your child attain his or her fullest potential, and become the man or woman he or she was born to be.

I wholeheartedly believe that playing sports is a good thing for every child. Children need to engage in physical activities as they grow to help them develop well. However, there are certain types of physical activities that are not good for your child. There are *good sports* and there are *bad sports*. Bad sports damage your child's brain and prevent your child from becoming the man or woman he or she was created to be. As parents, it is our responsibility to keep our children away from all such harmful, unhealthy activities, no matter what they are.

Healthy sports will protect and aid your child's brain development, helping your child become more intelligent by honing spatial awareness, mental and physical agility, while providing a sense of pride in being an integral part of a team, or setting and achieving a personal goal. Bad and unhealthy sports, on the other hand, will damage your child's brain and make your child less intelligent, keeping him/her from exploring and achieving all they were meant to be.

What are bad/unhealthy sports?

They are the high-impact, high-contact sports such as:

- Football
- Ice hockey
- Rugby
- Mixed martial arts
- Boxing
- Wrestling

In these types of sports your child suffers repeated blows to the head in every play, which cause brain damage.

What are good/healthy sports?

They are non-contact sports such as:

- Swimming
- Basketball
- Baseball/Softball
- Track and field sports
- Volleyball
- Badminton
- Lawn Tennis
- Table Tennis
- Golf
- Squash

While every sport has some level of potential injury, in these types of sports your child does not suffer repeated blows to the head in every play. Your child's brain is protected.

Since 1957 doctors have told us that the bad/ unhealthy sports I have just listed have no place in the lives of children and in school or recreational programming. Today, doctors continue to confirm that there is no reason whatsoever why a child should be allowed by a parent to play bad/ unhealthy sports, which have been proven to be too dangerous for children.

I believe that children should be encouraged to play the healthier, non-contact sports. Parents can visit the website of the International Olympics Committee (https://www.olympic.org/the-ioc) to view a list of the safer sports they should engage in and enjoy. Of course, when children play these non-contact sports, there is still a risk of suffering accidental injury. Accidents do occur, and players can suffer accidental injuries. However, blows to the head and intentional injuries of our brain and bodies do not occur in every play of a non-contact sport, unlike the high-contact ones. In the healthier sports, intentional injuries are not needed for the play and are not intrinsic to the game. Even though they are by design, healthier, we still must play non-contact sports with child safety in mind, and ensure that they are strictly regulated and supervised. Unsportsman-like behavior, and aggressive and violent tactics and plays must also be discouraged by penalties and/ or dismissal from the game.

As a modern society, whenever we identify a potentially dangerous activity or situation, we protect our children from it. Dangerous, physically risky activities should be left only for adults above the age of 18, who have reached the age of consent. The age of consent is biologically and developmentally appropriate, because a child's brain becomes the brain of a fully developed adult between the ages of 18 and 25 years old. Adults who wish to play bad/unhealthy sports can choose to play at their own risk—but not children.

The Age of Consent

In the United States, the typical age of consent is 18 years old, when a child becomes a legal adult. In most states, children cannot purchase cigarettes until they are 18, or legally drink alcohol before they turn 21. Our children are also legally restricted from engaging in potentially dangerous activities like skydiving, deep-sea diving, car racing and smoking marijuana, in order to protect them.

We do not let children join the armed forces until they are 18. We do not let children vote until they are 18. At this time, developmentally speaking, a child's brain has matured enough that they can understand the ramifications and consequences of his or her decisions and actions.

I will be the first to stand by every adult over the age of 18 to fight and defend his or her right, freedom, freewill and liberty to play any sport they want to play. Adults should be free to do whatever they wish as long as their choices do not pose any danger or threat to the life of another human being. That adult also must be made aware of the potential dangers and risks involved in the potential activity they are considering. No one should be deceived, as deception limits the freedom of the individual to make the best and/or healthiest choice possible.

However, when it comes to a child, I will also be the first to stand by every young person below the age of 18 to fight and defend the right, freedom, freewill and liberty of every child to be protected from harm.

Likewise, we as parents should keep potentially dangerous sports away from our children and protect them from brain damage. Your child's brain is what gives him/her emotional stability, academic intelligence, the ability to make rational decisions and solve complex problems, be a lifelong learner, feel emotions, display empathy, be a good friend and a respectful, loving future spouse and parent. In essence, the brain gives life. As a result, it absolutely must be protected, nourished, and cherished at all cost.

In the following pages, I will share with you more heartbreaking instances, like Dan's tale, in which the brain was not protected or cherished—to the peril of the individuals, and their families.

2

It's Crazy to Tell Me That My Child Should Not Play Football

One of the most difficult things I have struggled with in my life as a physician and as a Christian is the truth. The truth can get me very angry, flustered, disappointed and depressed. But one of the greatest lessons I have discovered in my career and in my faith journey is that even though truth is always inconvenient, I cannot deny it. Come what may, the truth will always prevail. It may take a long time to prevail, but when it prevails I will want to be on the side of the truth.

Despite truth's inconvenience, when we embrace it for what it is, we enlighten and empower ourselves to become better individuals. The impossible shall begin to become possible. We must not fall to the temptation to avoid the inconvenience and difficult lessons of the truth, and create our own alternative truths that are convenient for us. Convenient alternative truths can only lead us into great darkness, which I have witnessed too many times in the diseased brains of individuals I have examined, and in the lives of parents and families who have been destroyed because of a loved one's brain damage —the sad result of playing contact sports.

I fully understand the inconvenience and difficulty parents face when a physician like myself advises them that their children should be kept away from football and other types of contact sports—activities they may like and excel in. I hope you understood my heart about this. Our children have played football across the centuries and it was accepted tradition and practice. In fact, it was and remains a way of life for many communities in the United States. Communal life in many communities across the United States is centered and continue to be centered around football. This has been an accepted and celebrated way of life and culture, but please allow me to explain it in another way.

Let's say you have a 10-year-old son who has seen his friends smoke cigarettes behind the stadium after school. They're the cool kids, and your son wants to continue to fit in with this crowd. He comes to you and asks if you would allow him to have just one cigarette to take with him to school so he can smoke it with his buddies. What would you do as a parent? I believe all parents would say a bold "NO!" And why would a parent say no? Simply, because tobacco and nicotine products have been proven to be harmful, addictive, and unhealthy—for anyone, of any age—especially children.

If we would not allow a 10-year-old child to smoke even one cigarette, why would we then place a helmet on the head of that child, send him to a field and make him suffer many blows to his head in only one game of football? Do you know that a child can suffer more than 50 blows to the head in only one game of football? Each violent blow to your child's head causes injuries to your child's brain. These injuries are known as sub-concussions and concussions. These are injuries to your child's brain, and they are permanent.

So, let us step back for a moment, take a deep breath and ask a question. Which is more dangerous, one cigarette or a concussion of your child's brain? Of course, a concussion of your child's brain is more dangerous than one cigarette.

If a concussion is more dangerous than one cigarette, why then would parents across the United States, and the world, continue to intentionally expose their children to the risk of permanent brain damage by allowing them to play unhealthy sports that include football, ice hockey, rugby, mixed martial arts, boxing, and wrestling? Why would parents call me crazy (and worse, I'm sure) for suggesting that they stop exposing their children to brain damage? I am not the one who is crazy. Our modern society may be, though!

The first time parents reacted angrily towards me when I advised that they should immediately remove their child from playing football in school, I was deeply saddened. I could not understand why they reacted so heatedly especially when I meant well. I began to study this pattern of behavior in an attempt to figure it out.

Without knowing it, the way we think, our beliefs, our perceptions of the environment, and every aspect of our intelligence as individuals have been permeated, influenced and controlled by all forms of print and social media, corporate marketing, companies that manufacture and sell products, television shows and news programs, and the sports and entertainment industries. We may want to believe that we are independent individuals who have the freewill and liberty to think and do whatever we want to do, especially in the United States of America. This may be very far from the truth and reality.

The reality is that as individuals the way we think forms beliefs. Our minds are controlled by expectations, traditions, norms and cultures of society that have been set and determined by the information fed to us over time. Over the decades and centuries, we have been told, and have come to believe that a child must play football. Depending on where you may live, you may believe that you must, and have to do something to feel whole, to have a sense of belonging in your community, and to feel fulfilled and accepted. For instance, if you live in Ireland or Australia, you may believe that your child must play rugby. If you live in Canada, you may believe that your child must play ice hockey. These are all good, but stop for a moment, take another deep breath and think: *Says who? Why?*

Once your mind becomes embedded in these expectations of society, you are more likely to become tribal and emotional in your thinking and less able to see things as they really are (by "tribal", I mean engaged in "group-think" or thinking what everyone else does). You may begin to deny, ridicule or dismiss any alternative perspective that may challenge the cast of your mind. Especially when that cast of your mind is not supported by honest, sincere and transparent scientific truths and facts. It becomes more expedient to lash out in dismissive anger and question the intent and good will of others who may not agree with you. I am guilty of this too. We all are guilty. This may be why you may think I am crazy for saying what I am saying. I am challenging the cast of your mind.

We must begin to free ourselves slowly from this zombie-like bondage and exercise our God-given free will to think and decide for ourselves as individuals. You have the power within you as a parent to think freely for yourself and decide what healthy games your child can play or not play. There is nothing wrong with doing the right thing for your child by refusing to let your him/her play unhealthy sports even when everyone else's kids are playing them. You are not crazy and Dr. Omalu is not crazy.

What may be crazy is, despite knowing what we know today, that our society will continue to intentionally, knowingly, expose children to the risk of permanent brain damage in unhealthy contact sports. If a child plays only one season of football, with or without a helmet, with or without suffering a documented concussion, that player stands a 100% risk exposure to suffering permanent brain damage. This includes your child. Yes, yours.

Is it not crazy that, as a society, we are ignoring these undeniable facts and truths of science?

3

The Brain Floats Like a Balloon inside the Skull

In the movie *Concussion*, Will Smith played me as Dr. Bennet Omalu and Gugu Mbatha-Raw played my wife Prema. About thirty-seven minutes into the movie, there is a scene where Dr. Omalu demonstrates to Prema what happens to the brain when a helmeted head suffers a blow while playing football.

When Will Smith was preparing for the role, we spent some time together so that he could grasp my personality, see my movements, and hear me tell portions of my story in person. It was also an opportunity for me to demonstrate to Will the science behind my discovery.

The demonstration seen in the movie is a direct result of the time we spent together. Will Smith, who is one of the most intelligent people I have met, actually came up with the demonstration himself. He wanted to develop a mental picture so he could fully understand how the brain suffers serious damage even when a player wears a helmet and the skull, face, and scalp remain free from any fracture or injury.

Before I explain the demonstration, it will be helpful for you to know that the brain sits cradled inside the human skull without being attached to the skull. There are big spaces inside the center of the brain called ventricles, which are like balloons, but do not contain air. These ventricles give the brain some measure of buoyancy. This buoyancy, however, is not designed to fully cushion the brain.

At the start of the experiment, Will and I found a big transparent cylindrical glass jar with a lid that could be clamped to the jar. We added about 1 teaspoon of clean tap water to represent the thin film of fluid on the brain inside the skull called cerebrospinal fluid [CSF]. We filled a rubber balloon with tap water to give it some weight, and then inflated the rubber balloon so that it was large enough to be placed inside the glass jar without touching the walls. We tied the tip of the balloon, placed it inside the jar, and clamped the lid closed. We then lifted the glass jar from the table while holding it with two hands and shook the glass jar back and forth. While doing so, we watched what happened to the balloon. As someone held the jar containing the inflated balloon, another person also firmly struck it with the palm of the hand—but not violently enough to break the jar. Again, we watched to see what happened to the balloon inside the jar. Of course, each time we shook or hit the jar, the balloon bounced around inside the glass jar.

The next thing we did was to wrap the sides of the jar with a thick cotton towel. The glass jar represented the human skull, the balloon represented the human brain, and the towel represented a helmet. We shook and hit the glass jar again and watched what happened to the balloon inside the jar. It bounced around inside the glass jar. We wrapped a second, and then a third thick cotton towel around the sides of the glass jar, and each time we shook and hit the toweled glass jar and watched through the top and bottom of the jar to see what happened to the balloon.

The conclusion was simple. One, two, or three layers of cushioning provided by one, two, or three towels that acted as helmets made no difference to the balloon bouncing around inside the glass jar as it was being struck. The more cushioning we added to the glass jar, the less the amount of force needed to hit the glass jar before the balloon moved around inside the jar. This is an illustration of what happens to the brain when the face, head or skull is hit, whether you are wearing a helmet or not.

While this homemade demonstration was not a scientifically validated illustration, it was an effective way to portray the concept to someone who did not spend four or more years in college studying the brain. And it was very successful, for after that demonstration, Will got it, as well as the film's director, Peter Landesman. That was my objective. I did not know that the demonstration would eventually appear in the movie. I know I am not biased in the least when I say that Will and Peter did a phenomenal job with *Concussion*!

Every blow to the human head has the potential to cause brain damage.

God did not create us and our human anatomy to engage in activities that cause repeated blows to the head. Our bodies do not have the capacity to withstand and completely tolerate them. Our creation and our evolution have not given us that capacity. Every blow to the human head has the potential to cause brain damage. There is no safe blow to the human head. The more violent and forceful a blow to the head is, the greater the likelihood of permanent brain damage. The more repetitive the blows are, the greater the likelihood of permanent brain damage. There is no question that repetitive and violent blows to the head will eventually cause permanent brain damage. We do not know the exact number of repetitive and violent blows to the head that will cause permanent and irreversible brain damage. However, we do know that only one violent blow to the head can cause brain damage. The brain can suffer permanent brain damage without suffering any diagnosed concussion while playing contact sports.

The brain is made up of about 60-80% water, and contains over 200 billion cells. It is an extremely soft organ with the consistency of jello or thick custard. Brain cells and fibers float in a sea of water; therefore sudden and forceful movements, forward or backward, or around the center of the brain can cause fragmenting injuries and disruptions of the brain cells and fibers. Once injured, the brain does not have any reasonable capacity to regenerate itself and cure itself completely. Research shows that there may be some cells (stem cells) in the brain that may be able to regenerate, but this observation remains only on the experimental laboratory level.

Each person is born with a certain number of brain cells. After birth, we can only lose our brain cells; we cannot create new ones. Unlike our skin, or liver, our brain has a very limited ability to heal and regenerate itself after every injury. The brain is an incredibly sensitive, delicate, and fragile organ. It reminds me of the youngest child in a loving family—the precious little one, who everyone watches out for, pampers, spoils and protects. Likewise, we have to protect our brains and treat them with the most delicate care. Losing one brain cell is too many. We should not engage in any activity that may intentionally kill even one brain cell. It is not worth the price. The brain is the seat of our soul and our mind. It is what makes us human. It is what makes us think, feel and express ourselves. It is what gives us intelligence, helps us relate to others, and helps us survive. I've said it before, but it bears repeating. Our brain is what gives us life, the greatest gift of all.

Balloon Brain Experiment

Materials

- Medium sized Jar

- 9-12 inch balloon

- Large towel

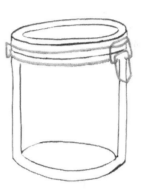

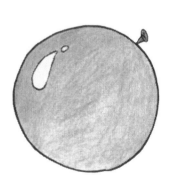

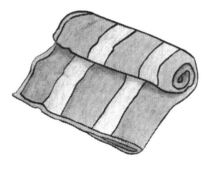

Continue to experiment ⟫——▶

Balloon Brain Experiment

Step 1

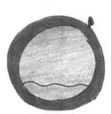

Fill the balloon with a small amount of water. Then inflate it to the size that fits within the jar without touching the walls of the jar.

Step 2

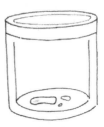

Place a few drops of water inside the jar.This will serve as brain fluid in this experiment.

Step 3

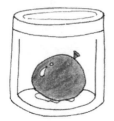

Place the partially filled balloon inside the jar and secure the lid.

Step 4

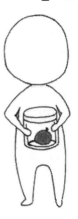

Hold the jar firmly and hit the jar with some force, observing how the balloon is tossed about in the jar.

Step 5

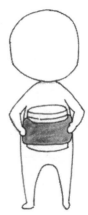

Now wrap the towel around the jar and hit it with the same amount of force and observe the balloon again.

Purpose

The balloon served as a brain while the jar was a head. The towel acted as a helmet that supposedly protected the head and the brain. Although from your observations you should see that there is no major difference between what happens to the brain with or without the towel (helmet) in place. A helmet does not protect the brain from moving around inside the skull and hitting the sides of the skull.

4

Myth: This $1,200 Helmet Will Protect My Child's Brain

Like the illustration in the prior chapter has shown, there is nothing we place on the outside of the skull that can hold the brain down inside the skull. So, a helmet on the outside of the skull, cannot hold the brain down inside the skull and prevent the brain from suffering an injury following a violent blow to the head. The helmet may be $5,000 or $50—it does not make any difference. Therefore the $1,200 dollar helmet you purchased for your child will not protect you child's brain, instead, it may even increase the risk of your child suffering brain damage! Continue reading—I will explain that explosive statement later in this chapter.

Those of you who are business owners, or those who have a business background, will understand what I am about to say. As Americans, we live in a free market economy called capitalism. People are free to do business. You and I are free to create a corporation and register it with the government. That corporation can create a product to sell or provide a service to sell. When a corporation sells a product or service, the intent is to generate revenue and make as much profit as possible, which is a good thing for the company. In order for corporations to sell their products or service, they must advertise what they sell. In order to advertise what they sell, a corporation often makes statements like: "Our product is the best in the market".

Says who?

But the law may allow statements like these. It may not be illegal for a corporation that manufactures and sells helmets to state that their helmet is the best in the market and is the safest for your child. All the corporation may care about is that you buy their helmet. You take the helmet, and they take your money. This sale drives their company's profits. The corporation is not in business to provide health education to you or your child. They are not in business to provide healthcare or injury prevention to you or your child. If you bought a $1,200 helmet for your child, it is actually very good for the helmet corporation that sold it to you. But is it good for you? Is it good for your child? Less likely.

Helmets don't protect your child from concussions or brain damage.

The helmet industry will be the first to tell you that a helmet does not totally protect your child from suffering sub-concussions and concussions. Helmets protect the skin and the skull and would prevent your child from suffering scratches, bruises and cuts of the face and scalp, and from fractures of the skull. Helmets may also protect your child from suffering bleeding inside the skull.

Helmets do not prevent sub-concussions or concussions. Helmets may simply reduce the risk of your child suffering catastrophic injuries that will result in the sudden and unexpected death of your child on the field of football following a violent hit. It does not protect your child from suffering permanent brain damage. If helmets did indeed protect the brains of football players and other contact sport athletes, especially when the NFL has the money to purchase the most expensive helmets in the market, why do we still have professional football players suffering sub-concussions and concussion on the field?

Helmets may increase the risk of your child suffering brain damage.

Helmets actually may increase the risk of your child suffering brain damage. It sounds counter-intuitive, but let us reason together. What causes brain damage following a hit to your child's head is the transfer of energy to your child's brain. Simple physics tells us that the greater the force of impact, the greater the energy transferred to the brain. If you increase the weight of your child's head by placing a helmet on his head, you increase the energy that reaches his brain. If you increase the size of your child's head by placing a helmet on his head you increase the energy that reaches his brain, especially when the size of the brain remains unchanged, while the size of the head with the helmet increases. If you place a helmet with a facemask on your child's head, your child will not feel any pain when he hits with his head. The absence of pain will make him more likely to lead and hit with his helmeted head and weaponize his head, increasing the number of blows to the head and the amounts of energy that reach the brain.

Many times, basic scientific concepts may sound counterintuitive and may not make common sense. But it turns out that a helmet, after all, may not be doing so much good for your child in terms of preventing permanent brain damage; which may manifest much later in life, after your child had stopped playing, and has long forgotten that he played. The symptoms of brain damage can begin to manifest in your child while he plays, months to years after he has stopped playing, and sometimes up to 40 years after he has stopped playing football, ice hockey, rugby, and other unhealthy full-contact sports with helmets.

What we think might be helping us might actually be destroying us.

My personal life has not been easy. I have encountered one challenge after the other simply by striving to do the right thing and applying my faith to my daily living. To cope with the stress, I have admittedly made poor choices. At some points in my life I have relied on drinking too many alcoholic beverages to help me keep on keeping on.

I had believed a lie—that drinking was helping me. At some point I discovered that it was a mirage. Spending so much money on brandy night after night was not helping me in any way. All it did for me was make me waste money. I could find other ways to help myself remain sane, while avoiding flushing my hard-earned money down the drain. At that moment I stopped this very bad habit, which after all was very harmful to my health since I developed gastroesophageal reflux disease as a result. So, I was spending so much money on something I believed was helping me but in actuality it was destroying me. Why am I telling you this story? The same principle applies to spending hundreds and thousands of dollars on buying helmets we believe are helping us, but in actuality are destroying us. I encourage you to stop, and see the light—just as I had to.

5

A Blow to the Head, a Sub-Concussion, and a Concussion

Let's go back to the movie *Concussion* and to the man I deeply respect and admire, Will Smith. At about 40 minutes into the movie, Will Smith (as Dr. Omalu) said, "God did not intend for us to play football." This is not just Hollywood talk. This is real. I have said this very same statement time and again, and will continue to. And yes, the structure and function of our bodies as human beings do not have the capacity to safely endure what games like football do the body of an adult human being, let alone the body of a developing child.

I believe that knowledge is power.

I am empowering you to know the truth about

head trauma, so you can make the best decisions possible for your children, and help other parents and coaches do the same. Understanding what blows to the head, sub-concussions, and concussions mean in the context of your child's health enables you to know the truth about what's really happening to your son or daughter's precious brain when they play full-contact sports like football.

When the head suffers a violent blow, and energy is transferred to the brain, the brain suffers three types of injuries that involve the microscopic skeleton of the brain cells and fibers, the walls of the brain cells and fibers, and the microscopic blood vessels of the brain. Microscopic bleeding occurs inside the brain. These types of injuries cannot be identified by a routine CT scan or MRI, which are frequently negative. Your child may suffer or not suffer any symptoms despite the injuries to the brain.

A **blow to the head** may be defined as a blunt force impact to the head. A **sub-concussion** may be defined as an injury of the brain, at the microscopic level, caused by a blow to the head without any immediate symptoms. A **concussion** may be defined as an injury of the brain, at the microscopic level, caused by a blow to the head with immediate symptoms following the blow to the head. It is important to know that sub-concussions and concussions can also occur without a blow to the head, when the head violently changes the direction of travel.

Please do not be confused. There is nothing mild about sub-concussions and concussions. These injuries are permanent and do not completely resolve in the human brain. Doctors have known this scientific fact since the nineteenth and twentieth centuries.

Whether or not your child has sustained a sub-concussion, or concussion, every violent blow to the head causes some type of injury to the brain. We do not have any specific threshold or cut off for what makes a blow to the head a violent blow. The key issue is that what may not be a violent blow in one circumstance for one individual may be a violent blow in another circumstance for someone else. Every blow to the head has the potential of being a violent blow; therefore, there should not be any intentional blows to the head, whether they may look violent or not.

There are so many factors involved in what makes a blow violent. What we may think is not a violent blow to the head may turn out to be a very damaging one in the long run, an injury that can cause brain damage, especially when the action is repeated over time. One violent blow to the head can cause permanent and irreversible brain damage. Several violent blows to the head can cause permanent and irreversible brain damage. Multiple violent blows to the head can cause permanent and irreversible brain damage. Doctors do not know when permanent and irreversible brain damage will occur. It depends on the individual patient. But generally speaking, the more violent the blows are, and the more repetitive the blows are, the greater the chances of suffering permanent and irreversible brain damage.

Following such injuries, the brain responds and goes into a state of change called neuro-inflammation. A parent may be told that his or her child can safely return to play after two to four weeks after a concussion. This may not be absolutely correct. Two to four weeks after a concussion, the brain has not healed and can remain markedly inflamed. The abatement or absence of symptoms does not mean the brain has healed completely. Any other violent blow to your child's head after he or she returns to play adds to the pre-existing damage and will increase the risk of permanent brain damage in the long term, many years later. When a child suffers a concussion, there is an increased risk of suffering a repeat concussion. And if a child suffers two or more concussions within a short period of time, there is an increased risk of sudden and unexpected death or catastrophic brain injury on the football field or after a game of football.

The safest thing a parent can do is to avoid intentional blows to the head of a child as much as we can. This will obviously reduce the risk of your child suffering any form of brain damage. Once your child's brain is damaged, that is it. There is no doctor who can completely reverse the damage.

The brain can become permanently damaged without your child ever suffering a documented concussion.

For every documented concussion, a person can sustain tens to hundreds to thousands of blows to the head and sub-concussions. Your child may play only one season of football, wearing a helmet, and suffer hundreds of blows to the head without one diagnosed concussion and *still* suffer brain damage—in just one season. The greater the number of seasons and years he plays, the greater the risk of exposure and the greater the likelihood of permanent brain damage. *Therefore, we should stop making it about concussions. It is about blows to the head, period.*

There is no other organ in the human body like the brain. The brain is a very special organ that behaves differently from all other organs in the body. The brain remembers every blow it suffers and all the resulting damage from that blow. Over your lifetime, beginning in early childhood, the brain accumulates all the injuries it has suffered from all the blows it has incurred. So over time, the brain suffers cumulative brain injury and brain damage, which can begin to manifest with mild symptoms. Over time, the symptoms may progress in severity and rob you of your life, like I have seen it do time and again with those who have played full-contact helmet sports. At some point (which doctors do not yet know) the brain resets itself after a certain level of damage, becomes self-destructive, accumulates bad proteins and begins to kill brain cells. The symptoms that may manifest over a period of years represent the disease called "Traumatic Encephalopathy Syndromes".

I have always been skeptical when I hear football experts and some doctors say that we can make football safe. How can we eliminate blows to the head from football? How can we make boxing safe and eliminate blows to the head from boxing? Let each parent ask these questions and decide.

Brains, especially developing ones, never heal completely.

The brain does not and cannot heal as well and as quickly as bones do. If a child fractures his or her arm or leg during a game, that child is immediately removed from play and is kept out of play for the entire season. The human skeleton has the capacity to heal completely without any persistent damage, especially in children. We would keep a child out of play for several months or more after suffering a fracture of his arm or leg, a fracture, which will heal completely. However, we would keep a child out of play for only several weeks or less after suffering a concussion of the brain, which will not heal completely. Unfortunately, our society has traditionally sympathized and empathized more with illnesses of our bodies that we can see, but when it comes to illnesses of the brain that we cannot see, we sympathize and empathize less. This needs to change.

The developing brain of a child becomes an adult brain around 18 to 25 years old. During this time, brain cells increase in size and develop hundreds of billions of intricate and delicate interconnections between hundreds of billions of other brain cells, while synthesizing and depositing myelin to cover the cell fibers.

This is a very critical time in the life of each and every one of us. I compare this time of development to the foundation phase of the construction of a 70-floor skyscraper. The successful, careful design and construction of the foundation is critical for the functional and structural support of such a tall building. There is a very intricate and delicate inter-connectivity between steel and iron rods and beams and poured concrete.

What happens to the brain of a child when his or her head suffers a violent blow is similar to what would happen to a skyscraper's foundation if an earthquake occurs while the foundation is being built. The intricate and delicate inter-connections between steel, iron and concrete would be disrupted and undermined. If the foundation is not re-constructed, (just like how the brain does not heal completely) and the construction of the skyscraper continues with the disrupted foundation, that skyscraper will not be as structurally and functionally sound as it should be when it is completed.

This is what happens to your child's brain. When a child plays unhealthy contact sports, the development of the brain, just like the foundation, can become disrupted and undermined and when the brain becomes an adult brain, it may not be as structurally and functionally sound as it should be, or was born to be.

6

Brain Damage in Football Is Real—as These Stories Illustrate

Over the years I have received thousands of e-mails and phone calls from parents who have shared with me the most painful stories of their children whose lives have been stolen from them by brain damage caused by blows to the head in contact sports. The stories I am about to share with you are based on true events and conversations I have had over the years, with names, specific details and circumstances altered to respect the privacy of those involved.

Todd's Story

One evening while I was promoting the movie *Concussion*, my phone rang. I had just checked into a beautiful hotel in Beverly Hills, courtesy of Sony Motion Pictures. The number kept calling—one, two, three times. Sensing the caller's urgency, I answered.

"I will never forgive myself," the man on the other end sobbed. I sat down on the hotel bed as the man continued to cry. I recognized his voice. It was a professor I had met many years ago at a conference in Philadelphia.

"Dr. Sullivan, why can you not forgive yourself?"

He said it was about his son—he ruined his son's life. I let him cry, not saying anything. Minutes passed. When Dr. Sullivan became sufficiently calm, he told me the story of his three sons. The oldest son, Todd, was the smartest of the three. In elementary school he exhibited intellectual abilities beyond those of gifted and talented students his age. All this young man did was read, read, and read. Todd was placed on an accelerated program for exceptional children and was given permission to skip several grades. In his first year of high school, he was offered admission to a combined pre-medical, medical, and Ph.D. program. He was set for life. All he had to do was to complete high school and enter college. With academics being a breeze, Todd had a lot of free time on his hands. And since he had never played any sport in his life, his parents encouraged him to get involved. They chose football because it was a rigorous game that would toughen him up and teach him discipline in preparation for the challenges of his medical and Ph.D. program. So they thought.

Todd played football for about two years in high school, and suffered several documented concussions. He left for college. The first year of his combined doctoral program was an incredible struggle, and for the first time in his life he began faltering academically. He simply could not cope. His grades turned from A+ to B- or C-. He dropped out of school, and took a year off to recuperate and rehabilitate. He enrolled into another college program, since he thought medicine might not be his calling. It did not make any difference. He eventually dropped out of school altogether and took a job at a local fast food franchise. He never completed college.

Understandably, Todd's parents were extremely upset and frustrated with him. In light of his bright future, and his previous demonstrated drive and ability, he was a total disappointment. His parents believed that he intentionally slacked off—there could simply be no other reason. They berated him, scolded him, and dismissed him, driving him out of the house in what they thought was a display of tough love. Sending him out into the world to find his own apartment and be forced to grow up seemed like it would knock some sense into him. The poor young man did not understand what was going on with him, or why his parents were reacting so cruelly. What had happened was that he had the *sense* knocked out of him. And I don't say that to be cute, or to make light. It is literally what happened.

The only thing Todd knew was that he never intended any of this to happen. He genuinely struggled and did not know why. It was only until the father saw the movie *Concussion* that they could put the pieces together.

As Dr. Sullivan was telling me this heart-breaking story, the poor man continued to weep on the phone, blaming himself. He asked me the dreaded question I knew was coming.

"So do you think that playing football damaged Todd's brain and made him less intelligent?"

I paused, carefully choosing my words. That quiet voice in my heart said to me, *Bennet, tell him the truth.*

And I did. I said yes. Yes, playing football damaged his son's brain and made him less intelligent. And that based on what we know now, even a single concussion can cause brain damage and make a child less intelligent.

Just like everything in life, some children may be more vulnerable than others. But given his son's story, I could not exclude his exposure to hundreds of blows to the head, with or without a helmet, and his concussions, as contributory factors to his academic struggles. And, I also could not deny that this type of damage may be permanent.

Why would an intelligent man like him, a leading professor in his field, not have recognized the risk of playing football, especially when it made basic common sense? That father may never forgive himself, but like Will Smith (Dr. Omalu) said in about an hour and 51 minutes into the movie *Concussion,* we must forgive ourselves, and we must forgive the football players, too. We might have not known any better then, but we do now. So what do we do with that knowledge? We cannot continue to deny the truth. And we need to be a part of the solution.

Patrick and Jonathan's Story

I met a man once, named Bill, who worked in the finance industry. He had a beautiful family: a lovely wife, two sons and a daughter. They lived in a gorgeous home in an exclusive part of town. But as we spoke I discovered that things were not as perfect as they seemed. In fact, he was living in a present-day nightmare, every parent's worst dream.

Bill was very troubled and had difficulty talking at first. His story meandered, as if he did not want to tell me the full extent of what had happened to his two sons, Patrick and Jonathan. He started out by explaining that his daughter, Chelsea, was doing extremely well and was in graduate school, but his two sons...his voice trailed off. He broke down and sobbed.

"Dr. Omalu," he wept, "I may have contributed to my kids damaging their brains."

I listened as he continued his confession, my heart breaking. It turned out that he had been a football coach in his sons' elementary school in his spare time. He had stopped coaching football two years ago. He could not do it any longer knowing what we know now and given what happened to his sons. It turned out that Patrick and Jonathan both began playing football at about the age of 6. Jonathan played until he was about 15, and stopped after he suffered a major concussion with symptoms that lingered for almost an entire month. His mother wisely demanded that he quit the team after that. But his older son Patrick played throughout high school.

Both Patrick and his brother, Jonathan, eventually dropped out of college. They could not cope and were not "college material", as he said. But it grew worse than that. His younger son, Jonathan, became a drug addict and abused narcotics including heroin. The older son, Patrick, who played through high school began struggling with depression, and did not respond to the prescriptions he was given. His mother found him in his room with a gunshot wound to his head.

The autopsy of his brain revealed Chronic Traumatic Encephalopathy (CTE). He was only 25 years old. The only person doing well in the family was the daughter, Chelsea, who did not receive thousands of blows to her head since childhood. For that, at least, the father was thankful.

After Bill saw the movie *Concussion*, he just could not forgive himself. This was why he stopped coaching football. He did not want any other person's son to be like his boys. I encouraged and consoled him, telling him that he was doing all he could do. He was acting on the knowledge he now has, and is actively spreading the message about the harmful effects of football on children's brains. In Bill, rather than pure pain, I see hope. He can teach all of us that we must forgive our past and embrace the limitless promise of the future.

The History of Concussions in Medicine

The stories I have shared with you illustrate what we have always known about all types of brain damage, whether it is suffered as a result of playing sports or not. Beginning with the Greek physician Hippocrates about 400 years before the birth of Jesus Christ, doctors throughout time have documented and reported the types of symptoms and diseases human beings may suffer when they receive violent blows to their heads.

After I discovered the disease I called Chronic Traumatic Encephalopathy (CTE) in the brain of Mike Webster (which I will discuss in a later chapter), I performed research for over six months, reviewing historical medical literature throughout history, all the way back to the time of Hippocrates. Every century has recorded the same conclusion: there is no safe blow to the human head.

What we know today about injuries to the brain is nothing new. However, over the years we have chosen to ignore the real truth and develop alternative truths that served our convenient ways of life as a society. Today, many of us in our American culture, both young and old, continue to pay the price for our alternative truths. We should stop, for what happens to one of us, even the least of us—a child—happens to all of us.

If your child plays any high-impact and high-contact sport your child has a 100% risk exposure to suffering brain damage.

Even one documented concussion can leave behind permanent brain damage that cannot be reversed. I said it before in a previous chapter, but I will say it again because of how fundamentally important it is. If your child plays football, ice hockey, rugby, mixed martial arts, boxing, wrestling and other unhealthy sports like BMX bike riding and bull riding, your child suffers repeated sub-concussions and concussions of the brain, which cause brain damage. These types of brain damage can manifest in significantly increased risks, sometimes up to a six-fold increased risk, for a variety of symptoms and diseases, in adulthood or as your child gets older to become an adult. These manifestations may include the following:

- Dying before the age of 42 years old especially from violent causes.
- Suffering diminishing intelligence, losing the ability to maintain long attention spans and acquire new knowledge.
- Dropping out of high school or college and not attaining higher levels of education.
- Losing impulse and mood control and exhibiting impulsive behavior to include the physical and verbal abuse of others.

- Engaging in violent, destructive, and criminal behavior, manifesting disinhibition including social and sexual improprieties, drug addiction and alcoholism.
- Suffering from major psychiatric illnesses including major depression, attempted and committed suicides, and other physically self-destructive behaviors.
- Motor and movement disorders.
- Memory impairment and loss of other cognitive and intellectual functions including diminished ability to engage in complex thinking and other executive functions, which can progress to dementia.

With all or some of these terrible possible outcomes, such a child is more likely to be less gainfully employed as an adult, is more likely to become a welfare or disability recipient, and is more likely to suffer diminishing socio-economic status and declare bankruptcy. Your child will be less likely to maintain and support intimate relationships with loved ones and families.

No doctor would know when the symptoms would begin in every child or which blow to the head will be the final blow that will cause permanent brain damage, which is why it is crucial for you as a parent or coach, to act now. You do not know how many blows it will take to cause your son or daughter's brain damage. The symptoms may begin while your child is playing, (without suffering any documented concussion) or after a documented one. It can even happen after your child has stopped playing, sometimes many years later, up to 40 years. The fact is, you do not know when it will occur. Take another look at the list you just read. Is it really worth the risk of your child's life and health to keep on as if nothing will happen?

Like my middle name says, there is no gift as precious as the gift of your child's life. Nothing, and I repeat—nothing—in our lives, not sports, not money, or the momentary glory of a few touchdowns, is worth more to a parent than the life of his or her child.

7

What Is CTE and How Is It Different From Brain Damage?

If you read *Truth Doesn't Have a Side*, you may have come across a statement I have made many times: "I wish I never met Mike Webster." I met Mike Webster on September 28, 2002, not in the way you would typically meet someone. I met him on my autopsy table. Mike changed my life. I lost my life that day, but I may have lost it for the good of all of us. I lost that simple life I yearned to live when I came to America on October 24, 1994. Instead, this discovery threw me into a tumultuous world that wanted to punish me for the truths I unearthed in my research. I won't get into too much of that story here, but if you want to know more about my challenges, and the faith that enabled me to overcome them, I encourage you to pick up a copy of *Truth Doesn't Have a Side.*

I've mentioned the term CTE in previous chapters. CTE stands for Chronic Traumatic Encephalopathy. In September 2002, three months after completing my training in brain pathology, I performed an autopsy on one of the greatest football players that had ever lived, Mike Webster. During that autopsy, I identified changes in his brain that I had not seen before. What I saw in Mike Webster's brain had not been identified in any football player before. In medical school I was taught about the brain damage that boxers suffered from, which was called Dementia Pugilistica. However, I was not taught about "Dementia Footballitica"! What I saw in Mike Webster's brain was not Dementia Pugilistica, and of course he was not a boxer.

How I named CTE

I showed my findings to other doctors in the hospital where I was trained and they confirmed that what I saw was real and had not been reported before. But before publishing the paper, I applied my knowledge in business management and in epidemiology (a branch of public health) and decided to give this disease a name. Like in a business, I thought that if someone discovered or developed a product, that person would give the product a name before introducing it to the market. But what name should I give it? I came up with three criteria.

First, the name had to sound sophisticated, sexy and exotic, so that people would like it, and would be more likely to use and say the name. However, while the name may sound sophisticated, it had to have a good acronym that would be easily remembered and pronounced even by a child. Secondly, the name should be fairly broad, without a very specific meaning so that if down the road someone else proved my concepts wrong, I would have wiggle room to exit and claim that after all, the name did not mean anything specific. Thirdly, the name had to have precedence, meaning, it must have already been used in medical literature as a descriptive term, but not as the name of a specific *disease*. This third criterion follows what is called the Daubert standard in the American justice system. This standard implies that for any scientific or medical evidence to be used in the court of law, it must have precedence and must be within the generally accepted principles of science and medicine.

At this time, I recognized that if this disease was truly what I thought it was, it would qualify as an occupational disease (which means a disease caused by your job), and it was a matter of time until it would end up in the court of law. And, oh yes it did—even sooner than I had imagined. Therefore, I could not give it any name I wanted, names like "Mike Webster's Disease," "Football Dementia" or "Dementia Footballitica", because I did not encounter any of these names as descriptive terms in previously published medical literature.

Over the months I carried out my research, I came across about thirty-seven descriptive terms for all types of brain damage caused by trauma to the brain. It was not difficult for me to select Chronic Traumatic Encephalopathy. It satisfied all three criteria. It sounds sophisticated and exotic. It has a beautiful acronym, CTE. It really does not mean anything specific, but stands for a bad brain associated with trauma that lasts a long time. It was broad enough for me. Finally, it already existed in medical literature.

Some people have told me that CTE is one of the most successful branding efforts in the history of sports medicine and sports, which is exactly what I wanted. I wanted the largest possible population to recognize the term and what it meant, because knowing both might save lives.

If you were to Google CTE or Chronic Traumatic Encephalopathy in September 2002, if you would have found more than several search results you would have been lucky. Today in 2018, if you Google CTE or Chronic Traumatic Encephalopathy—there would be thousands and thousands of search results. Simply unbelievable. I once visited my son's kindergarten class to assist the teachers, and most of the children in the class knew that CTE stood for some type of brain damage you may suffer if you play football or if someone hits your head. So incredibly impressive, especially at that age! CTE has permeated every fabric of the American psyche, even at the youngest levels of education.

CTE and brain damage have always existed

CTE and brain damage have always existed in everyone who has suffered brain trauma. It is a fundamental and primal concept in medicine dating as far back as the time of our friend Hippocrates. Some people recognize Hippocrates to be one of the first doctors who described and identified concussion as a type of brain injury and brain damage. Hippocrates himself called it "Commotio Cerebri," which in ancient Greek means "commotion of the brain." As I have said previously, over the centuries, doctors have confirmed in perfect unison that there is no safe blow to the human head. Blows to the human head cause brain injury, which results in brain damage, which is permanent. This is the fundamental and radical truth of science.

I was not the first to discover this concept for it existed even before I was born. However, the

Mike Webster autopsy taught us that when you receive all types of blows to your head, with or without suffering a concussion, with or without wearing a helmet, with or without manifesting any immediate symptoms, that over time, after you have received hundreds to thousands of these seemingly innocuous blows to your head, there is a significant risk of suffering permanent brain damage over time, sometimes up to 40 years after your very last blow to your head.

CTE is not the only type of brain damage your child may suffer when he or she plays unhealthy contact sports. It is only one of many. Unfortunately, America (and the rest of the world) has become too fascinated, if not obsessed, with CTE. This should not be so. The media should instead focus on all forms of brain damage that can be sustained as a result of playing full-contact sports. Your child can still suffer from brain damage without suffering from CTE. CTE is only one disease in a very broad spectrum of diseases your child may suffer when he or she plays unhealthy contact sports. CTE is also an advanced form of brain damage. Rather than focusing on CTE, we should focus more generally on all forms of brain damage.

The danger of unrecognized concussions

Take for instance, one Saturday morning, you innocently wake your son at 7:00 a.m., and have him brush his teeth and take a shower. Your son gets dressed in his football jersey and eats breakfast. Afterwards, you drive him to the neighborhood football field to play with his team. You hand him his helmet, help him strap it on, and send him out to the field to play while you watch, clap and cheer on the sidelines. At the end of the game, you help him remove his helmet, pat him on the back and drive him to a local ice cream shop so he can have his favorite ice cream (chocolate chip cookie dough with gummi bears on top). You, and every parent, should know that your son's brain as he is eating his ice cream is no longer as pristine as it was earlier that morning when he was brushing his teeth.

While he played football that morning, he received many blows to his head, sometimes up to 50 blows in that one game. Each and every blow he received was medically significant since there is no safe blow to the human head. Some of those repeated blows were violent blows, helmet on helmet, helmet on body and helmet on turf. At the end of the game, your child's brain has suffered sub-concussions and concussions. Most concussions go unnoticed and unrecognized. Mike Webster, in the 17 years he played in the NFL, allegedly did not suffer even one concussion!

A parent needs to understand that sub-concussions and concussions are types of brain damage.

If your child's brain suffers sub-concussions and concussions, especially when they are repeated, your child's brain is damaged. If a brain suffers a concussion, the damage has been done and there is no cure to reverse the damage. Taking your child out of play for several weeks and returning him or her to the team really does not make any difference. Removing your child from games and practice after a concussion only prevents your child from suffering further brain damage, catastrophic brain injury or sudden and unexpected death. No neuropsychiatric test will reverse the brain damage your child has already sustained. Making a diagnosis of brain damage in your child's brain does not reverse the damage. Thousands of years ago, Hippocrates advised us to first do no harm. He and thousands of other physicians throughout the centuries are still telling us the very same thing.

There is a broad spectrum of brain damage called TES.

As we discussed previously, the spectrum of brain damage your child suffers begins with the sub-concussions and concussions, and extends to other forms of brain damage and diseases like post-concussion syndrome, post-traumatic encephalopathy, post-traumatic epilepsy, chronic neuroinflammatory states, mood disorders, behavioral disorders, cognitive and intellectual disorders, memory impairment, motor and movement disorders, chronic traumatic encephalopathy and dementia. Some doctors have given this broad spectrum of brain damage the name Traumatic Encephalopathy Syndromes (TES). If you are curious about the definitions and symptoms of these diseases, I encourage you to look them up on the internet, on medical websites, in medical journals and research, which are widely available online.

CTE is only one form of brain damage but it is the one that has received and continues to receive the greatest attention. I must take this moment to emphasize that your child can suffer brain damage without suffering from CTE. The symptoms of brain damage may not be noticed until decades after your child, now an adult, has forgotten that he or she ever played football or other high-impact, full-contact sports.

What should I do if I think my child has brain damage?

All forms of brain damage, including CTE, can be diagnosed presumptively in a living patient based on the types of symptoms the patient suffers from. If you suspect that your child may have brain damage, you should immediately take him or her to the pediatrician. The pediatrician may refer your child to a specialized physician who knows how to diagnose and treat these types of diseases and symptoms. While there is no cure for brain damage, there are different types of treatments that can be prescribed for your child to control and reduce his or her symptoms. The best cure, however, is *prevention*: do not intentionally expose your child to the risk of repeated blows of the head in all types of human activities.

Early symptoms of brain damage

Some of the earliest symptoms of brain damage you may observe in your child may be:

- Subtle changes in personality and in behavior, inability to maintain focus and attention to learn.
- Inability to learn new things and recall what he or she already knew.
- Diminishing academic performance in school and in school work.
- Mood fluctuations and disorders including depression.
- Sensitivity to, and avoidance of a variety of sensory stimulations like light and sound.
- Movement disorders, instability, headaches and many other physical symptoms like fatigue.

There are a broad variety of symptoms your child may suffer because the entire brain is affected by sub-concussions and concussions. Every brain function can be affected and impaired. At the time of manifesting these symptoms, your child obviously is suffering brain damage or TES, but may not have CTE.

8

If Brain Damage Is This Serious, What the Heck Is the NFL Doing?

Around the world, wherever I go, parents ask me questions like this one. Everyone wants to point fingers at the NFL, the NHL, the WWE, the NCAA, Pop Warner Football and other sports leagues around the globe and blame them for causing brain damage in players, especially children. The easiest thing to do is shift the blame to another person, rather than looking inwards and possibly discovering that you may be the one to blame. This is not about the NFL or any other sports league. Let us leave them alone. They are not responsible for anything.

Earlier, I talked a little bit about America's free market economy and capitalism, which I love. I also love our free society. Again, in a capitalist economy, everyone has the freedom to do business, register a company or corporation, create something, sell a product or provide a service, and make as much money and profits as possible. It is a good thing to make money. However, I do not believe that the need to make money should override the common humanity that we all share. To me, one human life is worth more than the richest company in the world. Human life comes first and surpasses all things. Luckily, the corporations in the world that perform best and make the most money are the corporations that enhance our shared common humanity. Any corporation that may undermine the humanity of mankind will not last long. Short-term profits may look good, but the long-term sustainability of such a corporation will always be in doubt.

So, what do corporations do? Corporations sell products or services to generate revenue and make profits. The NFL and other sports leagues are corporations. The NFL sells a product, which is football, and provides a service, which is entertainment. The NFL is as legitimate as any other corporation out there, just as legitimate as corporations like Exxon Mobil, Apple and Facebook. They have the right to exist and do business. I want the NFL to make as much money as possible and make as much profits as possible. In our country, that is what good corporations have the freedom to do.

Can we and should we hold the NFL accountable?

As parents, we should not expect the NFL to take care of our children for us. That is not what the NFL does. As I mentioned regarding companies who make and sell football helmets, the NFL is likewise not in the business of providing health education or healthcare services. They are also not in the business of conducting and providing medical research. The last time they got involved in medical research, it was a disaster as expected. For example, in 2005 the NFL performed medical research and reported that the health outcomes of a child who suffered a concussion in a football game would be better if that child was left in the game to continue to play, than if that child was taken out of the game. This is bogus as expected, since medical research is not the service the NFL provides.

My point is that the NFL is not in business to raise your child for you. That is your job. The NFL cannot tell you how you can raise your child, nor do they (or Pop Warner leagues) compel your child to play football, same as the NHL, WWE and rugby leagues when it comes to ice hockey, wrestling and rugby respectively. The NFL does not force you to make your child play football. No one makes that decision for your child but you.

Since I performed the Mike Webster autopsy and identified CTE, I have never believed or hoped that the NFL would do anything about making football safer or educating the public about the truths of brain damage associated with playing football. And we should not expect them to do so.

Together, we need to be realistic in our expectations on what the NFL can do or not do. We cannot tell the NFL how to run their business. However, any corporation that does not conduct and operate business founded on real, radical truth, and instead goes by alternative truths it has developed, will not last long. It is in the interest of the long-term survivability of the NFL and the game of football in general that the NFL seeks and embraces the real truth in the way it does business. The real truth will always enhance and uplift our shared common humanity. Any denial by the NFL that football does not and cannot cause brain damage, is not good business, and is not the truth.

Recently, someone at a dinner reception asked me what I would do if I were the commissioner of the NFL. I did not have to even think. I responded that I would immediately issue a public statement with the stance that playing football is a potentially dangerous activity like many other dangerous activities in our lives, but that it is an absolutely fantastic game. I would elaborate by saying that if you choose to play, there may be a risk of suffering injuries including brain injuries.

Period. That is the truth.

Can you imagine what goodwill this short but honest statement would bring to the NFL? Such a simple truth will no doubt enhance the brand identity and value of the NFL and improve public trust. *The simplicity of the truth can even be more fantastic and more beautiful than football.*

9

Should Football Be Banned to Protect Our Children?

No, football should not be banned. I have never vouched for the banning of football. Nothing should be banned in a free society like ours. There will always be dangerous activities in a free society. Such dangerous activities and factors should not be banned but must be adequately regulated. Take for instance smoking cigarettes, drinking alcohol, deep-sea diving and skydiving; these are dangerous activities, but they have not been banned. They have been regulated. The most frequently encountered regulation in our free society is the protection of our children. We protect our children from all forms of danger-ous activities and pass laws to ensure they are protected. We do not leave this protection to the mercy of the individual parent.

After their most admirable position in 1957 that children should not play unhealthy sports, the best doctors for children in the United States, and now in Canada, came out again in 2011 to advise that every doctor must encourage children to participate in healthy sports in which intentional blows to the head are not central to the game.

A game is meant to be recreational, rejuvenating and invigorating for our bodies. When a game deviates from this, it becomes physically destructive and debilitating, and is no longer healthy. Putting the past behind us and moving into the future with great hope and promise, we can, and should, create new games for our children to play, new games that are both exciting, safe and healthy, games that may even be more fantastic than football as we play it today. Yes, we can do it, if we collectively come together as one society in agreement.

Rather than banning games, we should create new and improved ones. As humans in an ever-changing world, we must adapt to these changes to ensure the future of humanity. The good thing is that as we become more intelligent and enlightened, we will gladly give up the obsolete ideas and the ways of our past to embrace the forward thinking of the present and the future. Mankind of 2018 is obviously more intelligent than mankind of 1718, 1818 or 1918. We have greater and faster access to information and can analyze data at rates that were deemed sheer fantasy less than 100 years ago. The Mike Webster autopsy was a turning point in this evolution. On September 28, 2002, we saw a great light in our understanding of brain injury and brain damage in sports. Our lives were changed by Mike Webster. Science and faith revealed the radical truth to us and we evolved. We are now more intelligent in the ways we perceive and understand sports and brain damage. We have to apply this greater intelligence to the way we live our lives.

We cannot continue to live in the darkness of our past. This is not who we are as Americans. Any subculture that refuses to progress and advance along with mankind unfortunately will be left behind. If you don't believe it, I encourage you to consider the now-defunct Blockbuster Video, a company that had dominated the video rental industry when I was in medical school nearly 30 years ago. Where are they today? They are no longer in business, because they refused to see the future, and adapt to it. We do not want the same to happen to the games we love so much. Football and other unhealthy contact sports must evolve with society; otherwise they will be left behind and become a thing of the past.

Your belief is no different from mine: no child deserves to suffer brain damage from repeated blows to the head while playing a game. I know that one person can make a difference and begin to change the world. I am not that one person. It is you who is reading this book. Change for our children can begin with you and can come from you. All you have to do is stand up and speak out clearly and quietly on what you believe. The unhealthy games we play need to change.

10

Is It Child Abuse If I Let My Child Play Football?

As I discussed in the last chapter, our society evolves naturally. Although we may not realize it, we change over time. Consider the recent past: decades ago in our country, people of color were not allowed by law to marry outside of their demographic. This changed when several individuals unified, stood up for the truth, and spoke out for our shared common humanity. They challenged all of us and changed the law. In the recent past, the law did not allow minorities to move around freely and attend schools and other institutions they wanted to attend. In the fullness of time, this was changed when several individuals, again stood up for the truth, spoke out for our shared common humanity, challenged all of us and changed the law. Change is a good thing. Change makes us a better people. We should not be afraid of change; both in the way we think and in the way we live our lives.

In society, we may choose to live our lives in certain ways and hold onto certain belief systems for a very long time. At some point, we may have to change our belief systems, as we, as humans, become more intelligent and more knowledgeable. Something that seemed alien, uncomfortable, or unfamiliar in the past may indeed become accepted traditions today and in the future. There is nothing wrong with that.

What is child abuse?

In order to maintain my license as a physician, I have to attend child abuse classes and receive certification in recognizing and reporting any type of child abuse that I witness. The basic and fundamental definition of **child abuse** *is the intentional exposure of a child to a known risk of injury.* A physical injury does not have to occur to qualify as child abuse or neglect, or child endangerment. For example, you can leave your seven-year-old child home alone on a Friday night and go clubbing with your friends, and your neighbor may notice that your child is home alone and calls the police. The police may issue a warning to you and tell you never to do that again. If the next Friday you repeat the same thing and another neighbor calls the police, you may lose the custody of your child although your child has not suffered any injury. If you give your ten-year-old child a beer at a restaurant, someone at the restaurant may alert the police and you may be arrested for abusing or endangering your child for giving your child an illegal and harmful substance. There was a time when giving a child alcohol to drink may have been accepted by different societies across the world, but with the knowledge gained from the evolution of science and technology, we now have collectively determined that giving children alcohol is harmful and damages the development of their brains.

Is making a child play a sport that has repeated blows to the head child endangerment?

My answer is yes. I believe that knowing what we know today, beginning with the Mike Webster autopsy more than fifteen years ago, intentionally making a child play a sport that has a 100% risk exposure to brain damage, in which that child suffers repeated blows to his or her head in every play of the sport, may qualify as child abuse or child endangerment. Again, the intentional exposure of a child to a risk of injury is the very definition of child abuse. With this knowledge, a parent who sends his child to play football, and that child is injured, if that is not child abuse, what is?

I have attended numerous medical and scientific conferences around the world. In several of these conferences, I have discussed this issue as a panelist alongside other physicians and parents. While most parents agree with my position, however, many have said that while this may be true, we should not phrase it that way because saying that allowing a child to play football or any full-contact sport is child abuse is not convenient or politically correct, and it may offend some people. I beg to differ.

Social media and the internet, while good for keeping connected with the world around us in positive ways, has a dark side. Many of us have allowed these forms of communication and connectivity to influence us and perpetuate lies that control our hearts and minds, and ultimately, cause great harm to us, and our children. There is now a pervasive and emerging battle between the real truth and alternative truth. Prior to the internet, propaganda and alternative truths could be spread by controlling the media, controlling what is printed in newspapers and magazines and what is said on radios and televisions. There was a geographic restriction and limit to the number of hearts and minds that could be reached in a limited amount of time. The internet has removed these restrictions and limits. At the click of a tab on a computer, hundreds of millions of people, hearts and minds can be reached at an instance with an alternative truth that is simply a falsehood with some type of agenda and objective to undermine the real truth and control the hearts and minds of people. If this falsehood is sustained and fed through social media and the internet it can eventually displace the real truth to become accepted as the truth. There is a danger that society will begin to recognize and accept alternative truths as real truths for the convenience of a minority of us who seek control of society, our hearts and our minds. We must recognize this threat and battle for what it is. Convenient alternative truths and political correctness will not save your child's health or wellbeing. In fact, in this context, it is your child's enemy.

We must recognize this threat and battle for what it is. There can only be one truth. Truth doesn't have a side; truth doesn't have an alternative. If we begin to blur the truth, we begin to seek alternative narratives in order to serve our convenience. With alternative truths we can only develop false solutions and not real, true, lasting and sustainable ones. In doing so, we will lead ourselves to a deep abyss of darkness and destruction.

The truth today is that if your child plays a harmful contact sport like football, your child is more likely than not to suffer some type or some degree of brain damage. Knowing what we know today, if you ignore this truth, and intentionally expose your child to this known risk of injury, are you not endangering your child? It is a very simple question each and every parent has to answer.

Playing full-contact sports prevents children from acheiving their optimal potential.

Dr. Amir Sariaslan and his research colleagues in England, the United States and Sweden reported in 2016 that traumatic brain injury suffered by children under the age of 25 years old causes a substantial economic impact on the rest of our society. Surprisingly, there is a cumulative cost of about $1.1 trillion dollars on the United States economy over 30 years caused by lost productivity alone because of the brain damage children have suffered from exposure to head trauma. This is only about lost labor productivity alone. They did not consider the cost of health care, health monitoring, criminal justice and other types of cumulative costs. This is no longer something that should be ignored. Rather, it should be taken very seriously by all of us.

Statistically, people in the United States and Europe are having fewer children. Would we rather provide our precious children with everything they need to develop optimally and become adults that can compete with the rest of the world, or do we want to expose a significant number of our children to the risk of brain damage in sports, undermine their ability to develop optimally, and be less capable of competing radically in the global market? This is a 21st century question we must begin to ask ourselves as a society. There are other types of healthy sports for children to play, which will help them develop their fullest capacities.

11

Should I Let My Child Play Lacrosse or Soccer?

There is a risk of suffering an injury in every activity we engage in as human beings. Even when we walk down the street, we may accidentally slip and fall. By nature, we do everything we can to protect ourselves and reduce the risk of such accidents. Instinctively, we as humans do not intentionally expose ourselves to physical harm or injury. This includes injuries of the brain. The way we approach choosing which sports our children should play should not be any different.

I have stated previously that there are many healthy sports to choose from, in which there are no repeated blows to the head or shearing injuries of the brain in every play. However, even in some of the healthier sports, there may be a high incidence of accidental concussions of the brain suffered by players. Soccer and lacrosse fall in this category. Yes, they are indeed lower-impact and lower contact than football or rugby. However, you might be surprised if I told you that soccer and lacrosse players may have the highest incidences of accidental concussions of the brain after football, especially in female players.

There are also other potentially dangerous non-contact sports that can cause brain damage although there might not be repeated blows to the head. These include BMX cycling sports, bull riding and any sport that involves bouncing and jumping, such as trampoline-based gymnastics. In these type of activities, there are repeated shearing injuries of the brain which over time, can result in brain damage. My advice to parents is that children should avoid these sports.

Lacrosse is the subject of fewer discussions and controversies because fewer people play the game and it is frequently (for right or wrong) perceived as an elitist sport in some regions of the United States. I have never played lacrosse and I do not know much about the game, but I will not advise any child to play lacrosse. Adults who are above the age of 18 can play, but children should not. Originally played by Native Americans, lacrosse is a sport that has evolved and changed over time. In the future, we can develop newer and healthier versions of the game that children can play.

Regarding soccer, many people around the world love and cherish this game. Outside of the United States, the game is called "football," not to be confused with American football. In order for us to truly enjoy this game of graceful footwork and speed, we must make it safer. Youth soccer game rules and regulations must change in this regard. First, there should be zero "heading" of the ball for any child under the age of 18 years old. Moreover, there is a greater risk of head-to-head impact when two players reach out to head the ball simultaneously. Using the human head to attempt to stop or change the direction of an object traveling at a relatively high speed does not in any way make sense in the 21st century. Second, no child under the age of 12–14 years should play soccer the way we play it today due to the level of player-to-player contact it demands. Like lacrosse, we need to develop newer and healthier versions of soccer for our younger children to play, a less-dribble and less-contact form of this game that so many people love.

As it is played now, soccer is not developmentally appropriate for children.

Soccer is a high-dexterity sport that requires advanced levels of coordination and synthesis of your central and peripheral vision, as well as positioning and balance through precise muscle coordination. The young, undeveloped brains of children have not yet adequately matured to exhibit these very high levels of adult functioning. If you go to a field to watch younger children play soccer the way adults play it, the first thing you would notice is that they tend to cluster around the ball and follow it en masse. They do not realize that soccer is a sport whereby each player has a specific position and maintains a specific position on the field in relation to other eleven players on the team. The eleven players on a team must coordinate their positions against the eleven players on the opposing team, who are also coordinating their positions as the twenty-two players play together to win. Younger children yet do not possess such high levels of spatial reasoning, coordination, and high-order thinking. Younger children also appear sluggish and frequently miss the ball when they attempt to kick it. At the same time, they bump into one another and fall. They always have to keep their eyes on the ball in order to kick it, and when they do, many times it's haphazard.

A soccer experiment with my daughter

I did an experiment at home with my daughter when she was about eight years old. I stood before a small soccer goal in our backyard and placed the ball about eight yards away. I asked Ashly to do a penalty kick, while I acted as the goalkeeper. She was very excited and teased me that she was going to score and win. "Okay," I laughed, telling her that I would do my best to prevent her from scoring. She walked about ten yards behind the ball, smiling very broadly. She asked me if I was ready, and I said I was. I had taken my position right in the middle of the goal as the goalkeeper. In a very joyful manner, she ran giggling and expecting to score a goal and beat Daddy.

She had her eyes on the ball while she ran. I watched her closely. When she got to the ball, she removed her eyes from the ball and looked up at the goal and at me, and kicked. Can you guess what happened? The moment she removed her eyes from the ball and kicked her right foot, she missed the ball! The power of her kick combined with missing the ball made her fall backwards. She was embarrassed and began to cry. I ran out to her, raised her, hugged her and told her that it was okay. But that is exactly the point.

Her precious developing brain had not attained the level of development whereby she could engage in such complex visio-spatial and muscular coordination. However, when I asked my son to do the same thing, when he was almost eight years old, he was slightly better than his sister. I wondered if there was any distinction between a boy and a girl when they engage in such complex sporting activities because of hormonally functional differences (before you stop reading, I'll explain more in just a moment).

Another factor that many of us may be sensitive to, if not offended by, is that of gender in sports. A longstanding question has been whether boys and girls or men and women at a variety of competitive levels, should play the same contact sports.

Let me begin by saying that it is a scientific fact that boys and girls are hormonally and functionally distinct. None is superior or inferior to the other. We are simply different. It is very important that you understand this. We have observed that in certain types of contact sports, girls may experience higher incidences of concussions and with symptoms failing to abate as quickly or as completely as in their male counterparts. The bold question we have to ask ourselves is whether we should modify some existing contact sports, or develop new types of contact sports that would be better suited to the physiology of young women and girls. Due to many factors, women and girls can be better at playing some types of contact sports than men and boys. However, we have to let women and girls develop the types of contact sports they want to play their way, on their own terms. Our society has been patriarchal for so long, and often we tend to view different aspects of our lives from only this perspective, while ignoring the matriarchal perspective. Both perspectives can co-exist equally. It is a good thing.

How soccer can be made safer for younger children

Getting back to soccer, I believe we need to develop healthier and safer ways younger children may play this game. For example, we may develop bigger, softer and lighter balls that may resemble smaller beach balls to make it easier to kick the ball. When this kind of ball hits another player, the hit may not be as forceful. We may also reduce the number of players on a field to decrease the risk of one player running into another. We may also have to make the game less about dribbling and more about passing the ball through kicks across the field to reduce the risk of player-to-player contact. Children can play this type of modified soccer until they mature to 12-14 years old at which time they would begin playing soccer as we play it today, but without the heading.

Shouldn't my child start playing sports as young as he/she possibly can?

Some people have criticized me, stating that if children do not begin playing a sport in early childhood, that it will affect their ability and expertise as adults, thus reducing the quality and excellence of play. I disagree with this position. Children do not join the American military until they are 18 years old. This has not, in any way, undermined the preparedness and readiness of the United States Armed Forces.

If a child begins to play American football at the age of 5 years old and plays through high school until he is 17 years old, by the time he turns 18 he will have played around 12-13 years and received thousands of blows to the head. There is no question that at this time, the child's brain must have suffered some type of damage to a certain degree, with or without CTE. That child's brain is no longer as pristine and capable as it would have been if the child had not received thousands of blows by the time he turned 18. This means that with such a long history of exposure, the child who has suffered brain damage will be playing at a much lower level of sophistication and excellence because of his compromised brain.

So, if we do not allow children to damage their brains while playing as children and allow them to play only when they become adults after going through intensive training, these children who are now adults are more likely to play with undamaged, better developed, pristine and more capable brains. As a result, these adult players would be more likely to exhibit unequaled excellence and attain levels of play that we may not have seen before in American football. There will be no harm in testing this model as has been applied to the United States military. We should not be afraid to do so.

12

Brain Damage Is Not Only about Sports

In my job as a forensic pathologist, I have been blessed to be a part of many people's lives. I've been able to share in their pain in some of the most difficult times they will ever face. I consider my job to be a calling to serve as a vessel of God's light, love, peace and joy in the darkest moments. I have seen mankind at its best, mankind at its worst, mankind at its lowest and mankind at its highest. Brain trauma can be a big challenge and the possibility of brain damage exists in every aspect of our lives.

On the autopsy table, I see so many more cases of brain injury and brain damage suffered outside sports than inside sports. These cases are caused by motor vehicle crashes, assaults, falls at home, falls in the street and accidents in the workplace. Injuries like these might be caused accidentally or have been inflicted by someone else. However, while I was studying epidemiology at the School of Public Health, University of Pittsburgh, I learned that a significant proportion of accidents could be avoided. We contribute to the risk of an accident occurring through our known or unknown actions and inactions. Our errors, actions and inactions are significant contributory factors to a high proportion of car crashes, industrial accidents and even airplane crashes.

For example, when you drive a car under the influence of drugs and/or alcohol, or choose to text while driving, if a crash occurs, it may not be an accident in the true sense of the word, because a crash is an expected outcome when you do these things and drive a vehicle on the road. This suggests to us that there are certain actions we choose to do or not do that may increase our risk of suffering accidental brain injuries and brain damage. We have to do all we can to reduce the risk of accidents in our lives.

Please, do not take what I am saying in the wrong way. There are still accidents that occur that are purely accidental—in the truest sense of the word. They happen in spite of everything a human being can do or not do to avoid one. However, as a society, we must continue to do all we can to reduce the risk of accidents occurring, and therefore, mitigate the risk of suffering serious injuries when these accidents occur. Even for natural disasters like hurricanes, we can always do something as a society to reduce the risk of human beings suffering injuries in natural disasters. The key issue is that we must not do anything intentionally that would knowingly expose any human being, not even one of us, to the risk of serious injuries especially permanent and irreversible brain injuries and brain damage. But this is exactly what we do in certain types of contact sports. This has to stop.

Some of the most difficult and painful experiences I have had in my career as a forensic pathologist have been with domestic abuse cases involving child abuse and spousal abuse. There is no justifiable reason whatsoever why someone should beat up an innocent child, hurt that child, cause serious injuries in that child, and even sometimes kill that child. It is simply evil. A young person can be robbed of his or her precious life by all forms of brain injury and brain damage suffered in the hands of a family member. As an adult, this child is more likely to live a less productive life, which may be riddled with violence, criminal behavior, drug abuse and never finishing high school. No child deserves a life sentence of condemnation.

There is also no justifiable reason for domestic violence in relationships. The violence of a husband or wife, boyfriend or girlfriend can cause serious injuries, sometimes brain injuries and resulting brain damage. If you are in any relationship in which your spouse or partner hits you, even once, you should seriously think of leaving that relationship. It has nothing to do with love and it is not worth it. Your life is worth a lot more than a relationship. You can always find love and another relationship elsewhere. Do not live your life at the mercy of someone else's conscience. Even minor hits, shoves and blows to your head inflicted by a spouse, domestic partner or friend can cause permanent brain damage over time, which can resemble the type of brain damage we see in contact sport athletes. Your life is yours to protect and no romantic love is worth your life, they are not even close. While you can always find love, you cannot find another life.

As a forensic pathologist, I have also encountered so many cases of what I may call foolish and irrational violence. Why would someone simply kill another person because of a fleeting moment of vexation? That person who has been killed is someone else's father or mother, son or daughter, brother or sister, husband or wife, niece or nephew who is very much loved and cherished, and would be sorely missed. Why would you cause so much avoidable pain to a fellow human being? The more I struggle to understand this irrationality the more abysmally confused I become. The inklings of an irrational mind may be understood only by the irrational mind. It is not for me to understand unless I were irrational. But where does that irrationality emerge from?

As a student of epidemiology, I discovered that a significant proportion of violent criminals and prisoners in the United States have had a history of exposure to traumatic brain injury and brain damage in their lives, especially as younger children and adults. The emerging question we have to ask ourselves as a society is whether these individuals with criminal tendencies and irrational violent behaviors may actually be patients of brain damage and not the evil criminals we perceive them to be? The sciences of epidemiology and sociology have long taught us that exposure to brain injury and brain damage makes it more likely for the patient with brain damage to manifest criminal, violent and irrational behavior.

These are challenging and deeply thought-provoking questions we must begin to address as a 21st century modern society. Do these criminals need long-term, rehabilitative and medical monitoring as the patients they may be, or do they simply need to be locked up in jails and punished like the wild animals we perceive them to be? The easier and convenient thing for us to do as a society is to lock them up, put them away and sometimes even kill them to punish them as a form of vengeance for the acts they have committed against society. What could make many a young American so irrational that they commit crimes as awful as murder? Could some form of brain damage from prior traumatic brain injury be a significant contributory factor? This is a subject we must explore further.

About seven years ago, I received a brain preserved in a chemical called formalin. It had been sent to me by another forensic pathologist. It was the brain of a military veteran who had committed suicide. He had fought in several battles in the middle east and had been diagnosed with Post-Traumatic Stress Disorder [PTSD]. The forensic pathologist had wondered if he may have been suffering from CTE since his symptoms before his death resembled that of Mike Webster and other football players I had published about. I spent my own money and time examining the brain. In those days I examined brains in my garage at home in Lodi, California. While my wife and young daughter slept peacefully, I would sneak out of bed around 3:00 A.M., drive the cars out of the garage and set up my dissecting table, instruments and water baths. I honestly did not know where I got that drive from, but I had to survive. Desperate problems required desperate solutions. I had been ostracized and labeled a misfit by my colleagues and peers in medicine; why, I honestly do not know. I did not receive any support from anyone, any organization or institution. But it is okay. Eventually I discovered CTE in the brain of this military veteran, and it was the first reported case of CTE in a military veteran who was diagnosed with PTSD. Since my paper, other researchers have independently reproduced and confirmed my initial findings. This, unfortunately, is an occupational hazard of joining the armed forces, training for battles and fighting in battles. Active military personnel are a high-risk cohort for brain damage. Many forms of brain damage are diagnosed as PTSD. However, I believe that not all forms of PTSD are pure psychological ailments. There are forms of the so-called PTSD that are caused by exposure to traumatic brain injury and represent actual brain damage. The brains of these patients who have suffered brain damage in the military and are manifesting symptoms may show a broad array of brain damage changes, which are permanent. Their symptoms may be progressive and permanent and are less likely to be cured by any form of psychological treatment or drug treatment. We have to do all we can do to research this further because active military personnel and military veterans are the finest of the finest of America.

13

I Understand, But It Won't Happen to My Child.

In my journey of sharing the truth about brain damage due to contact sports, an overwhelming majority of parents have been very nice and pleasant to me. However, there are parents who get upset with what I have to say, and disparage me in the strongest ways possible. Some even call me very ignorant and disrespectful names. I see and understand where they are coming from, and I do not get upset with them in any way. There are also the parents who are able to respectfully disagree with me, even strongly, and still continue to argue that their sons or daughters who play unhealthy contact sports will not suffer any brain damage. "It won't happen to everyone," they say, and will readily point out several retired football players or boxers who are apparently doing well.

I will concede to a degree and say that they may be right. But, please allow me to share with you an experience I have frequently encountered. Recently, I was at a public event in a small beautiful town. Everyone was very pleasant and lovely. One of the guests of honor and VIPs was a retired NFL player who had once been a very big star in a neighboring metropolitan area. He was a tall, good looking and elegant man. He was the center of attraction and everyone wanted to shake his hand, hug him, and take a picture with him. I watched from a distance. I actually liked him very much, for he seemed affable and full of life. It was apparent he was accustomed to the limelight, and handled the crowd with the excellence of an expert.

Because I was neither a guest of honor nor a VIP at the event, no one paid any attention to me. I moved around the venue, observing what was going on around me. I enjoy people-watching tremendously, and after a few moments I noticed a very attractive woman, probably in her late 30's or early 40's, staring intently at me from a distance. I initially thought that I was imagining things for why would such a beautiful woman be staring at me with my big belly! I chuckled and brushed it off.

After a couple of minutes, I caught her gaze again. I stared back at her, and she looked away. I became uncomfortable, so I left where I had been standing. She followed me. Finally, I stopped avoiding her, and I turned around and walked towards her with an outstretched hand and a big smile on my face. As I got closer to her, I noticed a very worried look in her eyes.

"Dr Omalu, I need to talk to you. It is very important," she said quietly, her voice shaking. I did not know who she was, so I was cautious. I preferred talking to her in the open, but she told me that she needed to speak to me in private.

"Please?" she said in a most compassionate manner, with tears in her eyes. I agreed, and asked if we could go to a more private location. Once we found a spot, tears began rolling down her cheeks. She introduced herself to me, and it turned out she was the wife of the famous retired NFL player outside.

I was not surprised. But I was rather stunned by the emotions she was expressing to me. Why was she crying? I held her shoulder and was cautious not to hug her since I did not want to be seen in a private place hugging a woman I did not know. However, I knew this was serious. My sense of empathy rose to the occasion and I trusted God with the conversation. I shut the door, hugged her, and asked her to sit down. She began to tell me her story.

The famous NFL player outside was not as controlled and collected as he made the public believe. In fact, in private, his life was falling apart and he was having major problems in his personal and family life. Only his wife and several close family members knew, but the public didn't—he had been able to deceive his fans for many years. She was almost at the end of her rope. Her patience was wearing thin, and she was on the brink of exasperation. Her husband was in denial of his escalating personal issues. He had become an alcoholic, could not remember things and was beginning to exhibit rampant fluctuations in mood with irrational outbursts of anger at the slightest frustration. He could not keep any job. They were about to lose their million-dollar home to foreclosure. While she felt privately devastated and very ashamed, in public her husband had made everyone believe that he was still on top of the world.

By the time she was finished speaking, I too, was in tears. I saw her as I would see my wife, my sister or my daughter. I felt extremely frustrated since there was nothing I could do. I consoled her, gave her my phone number and asked her to give me a call to schedule a meeting with her husband. I wanted to speak to him.

When he and I met, I referred him to a traumatic brain injury program at a university hospital where a physician who specialized in treating these types of brain damage could treat him. But the truth of the matter is, there was nothing I, or any doctor, could do to reverse and cure his brain damage. I encouraged her to keep on keeping on, that the retired football players I have met who are doing better than others are the ones who have very strong spousal support. He needed her more than she needed him, but he would not realize it because of his brain damage.

The absence of symptoms does not mean brain damage has not occurred

Over the years, I have had many encounters like this one. The lesson I have learned from these experiences is that you cannot judge the content of a book by its cover. Someone you may only know from a distance may not be who you think they are. I believe that every NFL player who has played professional football has suffered some type of brain damage to a certain extent, with or without CTE. However, not everyone will manifest the same symptoms to the same degree.

Some of us may be better at covering up, compensating for, and actually controlling our symptoms than others. And if there is an absence of serious symptoms that may affect the way you live your life, this absence does not mean there has not been some level of brain damage. And because we are all genetically different, the onset of serious symptoms may begin at a much later age in some people and a much earlier age in others. As I have mentioned before, it may take up to 40 years after you have stopped suffering blows to your head for serious symptoms to manifest.

For the same degree of brain damage, some of us may manifest the same level of symptoms, while others may manifest lower levels of symptoms. Some of us may even manifest higher levels of symptoms, in a range of negligible to severe. Brain damage behaves like most other diseases. For instance, a disease like hypertension or diabetes mellitus can manifest in innumerable ways in different people, yet it is one single disease.

Pointing out one or two retired football players who may be doing well does not justify your child playing football or other unhealthy contact sport. In nature, the 3-4% of us who are outliers may not behave like the remaining 96-97%. There is always interaction between genetics and the environment. Each person may be different in the way their bodies interact with their physical surroundings, stimuli, and potentially dangerous factors.

For example, five individuals may be exposed to the HIV virus, but only one or two may contract the virus, while the other three or four may not. It still does not mean that the five were not exposed to the virus, and it still does not mean that the HIV virus does not cause a dangerous disease when humans are exposed to it. It also does not mean that we should intentionally expose ourselves to the HIV virus just because not everyone who is exposed to it may contract it.

Permanently damaging your child's brain is not worth the risk.

Let's assume that your child was born with a brain that has the potential of performing at an A+ level of intelligence. Let's also assume that he plays an unhealthy contact sport like football for ten years, and receives thousands of blows to his head. When that child becomes a teenager or an adult, his brain may now be performing at a B- level of intelligence.

Unfortunately, no one would have ever known or suspected that actually his brain should have been performing at an A+ level of intelligence, but was compromised by the brain damage he suffered receiving thousands of blows to his head due to ten years of football. Before the Mike Webster autopsy, we never suspected these scenarios, but after the Mike Webster autopsy and what he taught us in death, we now know. And since we now know, there are no more excuses.

The guiding principle for modern society, especially for our children, is if there are known risk factors, our children must not be intentionally exposed to these risks. The single most significant factor in the causation of brain damage in contact sports is exposure to repeated blows to the head. We should therefore not experiment with the lives of our precious children by intentionally exposing them to these repeated injuries, waiting and watching to see if they will manifest symptoms of brain damage. It is not worth the risk. Unlike a car that has a spare tire, your child does not have a spare brain. Your son or daughter only gets one brain, and their brains are their lives.

But won't God protect my child from brain damage?

Despite knowing these risks, some Christian parents have told me that their children will still play contact sports. Instead of responding to these risks by removing their children from these harmful activities, they pray that God sends the Holy Spirit to protect their sons and daughters from brain damage. After all, like many Christians, they believe that God encourages us to pray constantly, and whatever we ask in His name, He will give it to us. Such a level of faith is a good thing, but also remember what Scripture teaches us. The Gospel of Luke, Chapter 4, recounts the story of the temptation of Jesus Christ after he fasted for forty days in the desert. Jesus Christ, who was filled by the Holy Spirit, was tempted by the devil, who asked Jesus to throw Himself from the parapet of the temple to the ground so that the angels would guard and support him from suffering any harm. Jesus responded in Luke 4:12: "You shall not put the Lord, your God, to the test."

Let us follow the words of Christ Himself and not put God to the test. If knowing that doing something, more likely than not, will result in a known outcome, why would we then do that thing and expect another outcome by asking God in prayer to alter the truth, thereby testing the faithfulness of God? God in His infinite wisdom knows why He created us the way we are and why we have evolved the way we have. The truths of nature must be adhered to. There are no alternative truths.

As a parent, when you are tempted to believe that your child will not suffer brain damage as a result of playing a full-contact sport like football, I encourage you to remember the facts. Any child, no matter who they are, who plays these type of games has a 100% risk of exposure to brain damage. The greater the number of years your child plays, the greater the risk of permanent damage. Boys who play football starting in elementary school, continue to play throughout high school and college, and who eventually join the NFL as professionals, have very high probabilities of suffering some type of brain damage to a certain degree, with or without CTE. Based on my vast education, knowledge, experience and research, I believe that upon retirement, 100% of NFL players have suffered some type of brain damage, to a certain degree, with or without CTE. May this truth empower you to make the right decision for your children.

A final word...

I strongly believe that together we shall do unimaginable things. Through faith, what seems impossible today will become possible tomorrow. But first, we must radically recognize the truth for what it is, THE TRUTH. There are no alternative truths, truth doesn't have a side and truth doesn't have a perspective or a prospective. There is only one truth and the truth can be inconvenient and can bring about pain. The truth can be extremely difficult and challenging. However, we must not deny the truth because of the inconvenience or pain it may bring. For when we deny the truth, we will lead ourselves into the great darkness of mistruths and whatever problems we may have will continue and will get even worse.

Simply said, there are no safe blows to the head of a human being. We must do all we can to avoid blows to our heads in all that we do in our daily lives. Yes, accidents do occur, but we must do all we can to avoid them. Intentionally exposing your head or the head of your child to even one blow should be avoided at all costs, especially when the blows are repeated and violent. Your child has only one brain and one life. His or her brain cannot be fixed once it is damaged. As I said before, the glory of a few touchdowns is simply not worth it.

America is the best society on earth because of our *freedom*. This is why I have written this book. I want you, the parent or coach, to know the truth. Knowledge gives us power and freedom. When you know about the dangers of brain damage in unhealthy contact sports, you can now reasonably and competently decide if it is something good for your child. It is your choice, and not the choice of anyone else. This is not, and should not be about what the NFL does or does not do. Even professional NFL players who are living right now are calling for the game of football to be changed, and for young people to know and understand the dangers of playing football. I challenge you to listen to their stories of how playing for decades has damaged their brains and harmed their lives. Again, you have the freedom, liberty and freewill to choose what sport your child can play or not play.

As parents, whenever we identify something that may not be good for our children, we do not experiment with it, we simply prevent our children from being exposed to that particular harm. Why should we treat football and other unhealthy contacts sports any differently when these types of sports are not good for our children? Children should play the healthy, non-contact sports that do not expose their heads and brains to repeated blows. When they reach the age of

18 and become adults they reach the age of consent to decide on what they want to do, or not do. However, I must warn that there is no age when repeated blows to the head may be safe.

The power lies within you as a parent to do the right thing for your child. Look inside you, and not outside, such as your neighbors, the parents of other children, or your community at large. The power and responsibility rests on you, and you alone.

With faith, courage and the light of the truth, we shall overcome the challenges we face today regarding brain damage in contact sports. Our first step together is a step you must take: do no harm. As you encourage your children to avoid contact sports, we in the medical field will continue to search for solutions, treatments and cures.

What I have shared with you has been for the good of you and your children. Speaking and explaining the truth has been my only goal. I care deeply about all of God's children. More than anything, I desire that every parent, coach and young athlete knows how to preserve their brains and therefore, their precious lives. Thank you for allowing me to share my often-painful journey of studying brain damage in contact sports with you. If you do not listen to Dr. Omalu, please hear the voices of the heartbroken parents and spouses who have watched their loved ones suffer and even die due to sports-related injuries that led to brain damage.

I believe that you can do the right thing, and that together we shall do the unimaginable.

Dr. Bennet Omalu
Stockton, California

Made in the USA
Middletown, DE
11 October 2018